The Carnivore Cleanse

A Revolutionary Approach to Healing, Detoxification, and Weight Loss.

© 2018 Alex Chase

Introduction

Despite (or more likely, because of) official dietary guidelines, people around the world are becoming more and more sickly.

Although overall life expectancy may be increasing - it is often at the price of more years of disability at the end. Even women, who are still expected to live an average of 5 years longer than men, *now only have the same number of active years as men.*[1] That means they spend those extra 5 years in poor health, often trapped in nursing homes and under palliative care.

Obviously the official guidelines are not working. Study after study shows that American are following those guidelines (less meat, less fat, more whole grains), and yet, 36% of us are obese, and 65% are overweight.[2]

The Organisation for Economic Co-operation and Development (OECD) estimates that 75% of americans will be overweight or obese by 2020![2] Diabetes, high blood pressure, heart disease, and other chronic diseases are at epidemic levels.

In search of health, or to kick start a diet, many people do a detox or try a cleanse. Usually this consists of some number of days where you only eat fruit. Or maybe a week where you only drink juiced vegetables, because this is what we've been taught is healthy.

Supposedly, this will remove toxins and/or heavy metals and give your body a chance to heal.

But these vegetable or fruit cleanses can often do more harm than good.

If you're a vegetarian for ethical reasons - STOP READING NOW. I completely understand and support your decision. You have my utmost respect. Seriously. Modern agriculture is wholesale destruction for the sake of the almighty dollar. Animals are straight up tortured and huge swaths of forest and grasslands are stripped to plant Palm trees for Palm Oil, or corn and soybean for the sake of cheap protein and deadly vegetable oils.

Although this diet/cleanse is carnivore - I support animal welfare through both action and money. We should strive to be humane always in our dealings with animals - even when those animals are destined to be food.

A portion of the proceeds from this book go directly to supporting humane farming practices.

That said, it is nevertheless true that humans evolved eating meat, and indeed, we have several dietary **requirements** that can only be met naturally through carnivore sources (vit. B, 9 essential amino acids, and Omega-3 essential fats).

If any kind of detox or cleanse is to truly heal the body, then these non-negotiable requirements for life must be available as part of the cleanse.

Not only are these essential vitamins, fat, and proteins not available through plant foods, plants have many natural defenses that are actively harmful when eaten such as phytates, lectins, and goitrogens.

You may think these concerns are overblown, but you can readily find studies of the harmful effects of eating too many plants. We'll discuss some of them later in the book.

So, what are we to do if we want to do a detox or cleanse and fruit and vegetables won't help us heal?

Certainly, eating clean foods and giving your body and digestive system a chance to sweep out unwanted substances is a great idea. More and more studies are showing the rejuvenating effects of both fasting (the ultimate detox) and elimination diets (an elimination diet is one where you eat only one food until you are free of symptoms and then gradually add other foods back into your diet in order to identify those that cause you harm).[3]

Paleo, Mediterranean, and high-fat diets like the Ketogenic Diet have become popular in the last decade because for many, they represent effective diets that can produce significant weight loss with less hunger.

They're also shown to reduce disease and help people live longer, more robust lives.

The Carnivore Cleanse is the Paleo and Mediterranean diets distilled down to their core - that essence which makes them so healthy and effective: Fish, Eggs, Beef and Water.

Prepare to discover what may be the fastest, simplest and easiest way to recover your health and kickstart a more natural and healing diet.

Welcome to the Carnivore Cleanse.

Join us online at:

https://www.facebook.com/groups/carnivoreplus/

How to Use this Book

1. Read through this book in its entirety to learn about the Carnivore Cleanse and how to implement it safely and effectively.

2. Decide how long a cleanse you're willing to do.

3. Pick a time to start - Try not to undertake a cleanse when special occasions or work responsibilities will create extra stress.

4. Download and print your shopping list.

5. Start your cleanse.

6. Evaluate the healing and benefits from

    your cleanse.

7. Repeat steps 2 through 6 as needed for

    additional healing.

Lets Get Started!

Problems with Vegetable

and Juice Cleanses

Because plants are not mobile and do not have natural physical defenses like animals (claws, tusks, speed, etc.), they've evolved to use chemical defenses instead (poison ivy and straight up kill-you-poison like most mushrooms).

Some of these defenses are chemicals which disrupt metabolism or digestion of essential nutrients. In this way they discourage insects and animals from eating them.

These chemical defenses are called "antinutrients".

Antinutrients are natural or synthetic compounds found in a variety of foods — especially grains, beans, legumes and nuts — that interfere with the absorption of vitamins, minerals and other nutrients. They can also interfere with digestive enzymes, resulting in poor absorption of nutrition.

And since humans are animals too, we are not immune from their effects.

Here is are just a few of the most common antinutrients that are found in fruits and vegetables.

- Lectins - found in bean, tomatoes, potatoes, and grains. Lectins bind to the sugar molecules called polysaccharides that cover the surface of most cells in your body. Just few raw kidney beans can kill you because lectins they contain can bind to the sugar coating on your red blood cells, which can make them form clots inside the blood vessels.

- Goitrogens - found in kale, broccoli, cauliflower, and strawberries. Goitrogens are substances that disrupt the production of thyroid hormones by interfering with iodine uptake in the thyroid gland. This eventually leading to swelling of the thyroid (goiter).

- Phytates - found in nuts, rice, wheat, corn, and soy/tofu. Phytic acid impairs absorption of iron, zinc, and calcium. When you eat high-phytate foods mineral deficiencies may develop over time. In fact, it may be a leading cause of anemia in developed countries.

- Oxalates - found in spinach, beets, nuts, whole grains, and berries. Consumption of oxalates may result in kidney disease or even death due to oxalate poisoning. The New England Journal of Medicine reported acute oxalate nephropathy "almost certainly due to excessive consumption of iced tea" in a 56-year-old man, who drank "sixteen 8-ounce glasses of iced tea daily" (roughly 33/4 liter). The authors of the paper hypothesized that acute oxalate nephropathy is an underdiagnosed cause of kidney failure and suggested thorough examination patient dietary history in cases of unexplained kidney failure.[4]

Beyond the antinutrients, vegetable and juice cleanses have other deficiencies as well:

- Low in fat soluble (A, D, E, K) and B vitamins. B12 is not found in plant foods at all and is required by the human body for energy production - not a good thing to be lacking while you're trying to detox and heal.

- Too much sugar. Fruits especially have been bred or genetically modified to have higher sugar content in order to make them sweeter. Vegetables like corn, peas, and potatoes have been engineered to have more sugar as well. Beyond just being empty calories, sugar feeds bad gut bacteria - NOT what you need when trying to heal.

- No fat. Omega-3 fats are *required* for life. Plants contain mostly Omega-6 fats.

- Low protein content. You'd need to consume a large variety of vegetables to get enough of all the essential amino acids required - and most of these are not the type you'd put into a smoothie regardless, for example: beans and lentils.

- Pesticides. Even if you're careful to get organic vegetables, they will still be covered in organic pesticides - some of which can be more toxic than synthetic.[5]

So we can see that vegetables and fruits are not the harmless superfoods we've been led to believe. In fact, in large quantities like we might use for a juice cleanse, they can be downright harmful.

While preparing for the Steve Jobs movie, Ashton Kutcher tried to follow Job's all fruit and nuts diet and landed in the hospital with pancreatitis - due solely to the overconsumption of fruits!

Thankfully, we have a much better solution!

The Carnivore Cleanse

A cleanse by definition is a cleaning, or a detox of the body in order to either kickstart a diet or perhaps to heal some illness.

People will also use a cleanse as a way to *stay* healthy. Maybe you do a cleanse every 4 or 6 months just to stay in vibrant health - which we think is a great idea!

But, again, in order to get any benefits from a cleanse, the cleanse must a) give the body the nutrients it needs to heal, and/or b) not add any insult to injury in order to give it a chance to rest and heal.

Now, the ultimate way to rest the digestive tract is through fasting. Fasting is one third of the Carnivore Cleanse.

Imagine a lion on the savanna. If she (that's right - the female lions do the hunting!) has had a successful hunt, then the tribe eats. If not, then the tribe will naturally fast until the next time prey is caught. None of this 24/7 snacking that we humans do. No 'revving the metabolism' by eating every 2-3 hours - which, by the way, has been proven to be a prime contributor to obesity and diabetes because it keeps insulin elevated which is a bad, bad thing.[5,7]

In fact, studies continue to show that short periods of fasting allow the intestinal lining to heal (healing issues such as Irritable Bowel Syndrome (IBS) and Leaky Gut).[8]

Slightly longer fasts (3 days) can completely reset and rejuvenate your immune system![9]

And, no, you won't waste away. Even if you're an athlete, fasting will not 'eat your muscle' - in fact, they actually RAISE your metabolism and increase growth hormone. Both of which support healing.[10]

But when you're not fasting what do you eat to detox and cleanse?

The trick is to eat a 'mono-diet' and find the simplest foods that provide the nutrients required for health with none of the antinutrients found in fruits and vegetables.

Several foods meet our criteria: Beef, Fish and Eggs.

Just take a look at how much more nutritious Beef is than so-called superfood vegetables like blueberries or kale:

(100g)	Blueberries	Kale	Beef	Beef Liver
Calcium	6.0 mg	72 mg	11 mg	11 mg
Phosphorus	12 mg	28 mg	140 mg	476 mg
Potassium	77 mg	228 mg	370 mg	380 mg
Iron	0.3 mg	0.9 mg	3.3 mg	8.8 mg
Zinc	0.2 mg	0.2 mg	4.4 mg	4.0 mg
Vitamin A	None	None	40 IU	53,400 IU
Vitamin D	None	None	Trace	19 IU
Vitamin E	0.6 mg	0.9 mg	1.7 mg	.63 mg
Vitamin C	9.7 mg	41 mg	None	27 mg
Niacin	0.4 mg	0.5 mg	4.0 mg	17 mg
Vitamin B6	0.1 mg	0.1 mg	.07 mg	.73 mg
Vitamin B12	None	None	1.8 mcg	111 mg
Folate	6 mcg	13 mcg	4.0 mcg	145 mcg

We will cover these in depth as we go along - for now just understand that these are complete whole foods that our bodies can easily digest, contain all the nutrients we need for healing and robust health, and contain little to no contaminants that might slow detoxification.

The third, and final component of the Carnivore Cleanse is water.

Beyond simply hydration, water helps flush heavy metals from our bodies and supports every critical step of detoxification. Unfortunately, our water is contaminated with all sorts of chemicals - antidepressants, fluoride, chlorine and more. We'll cover how to best to get clean drinking water in part 3.

So there in a nutshell is the Carnivore Cleanse.

If you're not eating a meal - Fast and let your body rest.
If you're hungry - Eat Meat and let your body heal.
When you're thirsty - Drink Water and let your body detox.

I told you it was simple. Now, let's dive into the details!

Carnivore Cleanse Part 1: Fasting

Fasting is the willing abstinence or reduction from some or all food, drink, or both, for a period of time.

People become very stressed at the mention of fasting when, in fact, we all do it daily.

Breakfast literally means the meal which 'breaks the fast' - typically eaten in the morning but could apply to the first meal of the day regardless of when it's eaten. So every night you fast for maybe 8-12 hours between dinner and breakfast.

Some people only eat one meal per day while on a cleanse. In that case simply fast until you have your one meal.

There are many ways to Fast but for the Carnivore Cleanse we really only recommend 3 types.

Type 1: Intermittent Fasting.

Intermittent fasting is simply extending the fast until later in the day. Skip 'breakfast' and have lunch as your first meal and you've extended your fast to 16 hours. That is 4 additional hours where you're burning excess body fat (which is where a lot of toxins are stored) for energy and you're giving your digestive tract more time to rest and heal.

And more and more studies continue to come in with positive findings for intermittent fasting
- Early Time-Restricted Feeding (skipping breakfast) Improves Insulin Sensitivity, Blood Pressure, and Oxidative Stress Even without Weight Loss in Men with Prediabetes.[11]
- Intermittent Fasting (IF) is reported to improve the lipid profile; to decrease inflammatory responses, reflected by changes in serum adipokine levels; and to change the expression of genes related to inflammatory response and other factors. Studies on obese individuals have shown that patient compliance was greater for IF than other traditional nutritional approaches

(calorie restriction), and IF was found to be associated with low oxidative stress. Recent reports suggest that IF exerts a positive impact on the metabolic derangements commonly associated with cardiovascular diseases, and that it may be a viable and accessible intervention.[12]

- In a series of case reports, a lifestyle intervention that included daily short-term fasts was able to significantly improve Alzheimer's symptoms in 9 out of 10 patients.[13]

And finally, most importantly for the purpose of our cleanse:

- When we fast, the cells in the body initiate a cellular "waste removal" process called autophagy. This involves the cells breaking down and metabolizing broken and dysfunctional proteins that build up inside cells over time. Increased autophagy may provide protection against several diseases, including cancer and Alzheimer's disease.[14,15,16,17]

If you want to try fasting, Intermittent Fasting is the way to start. Simply delay your first meal until Noon. Or just don't eat at all until you're hungry (which may not be until dinner, or even the next day!) and know that skipping those meals is actually very healing.

Intermittent fasting can be done on a daily basis.

Type 2: 24 Hour Fasts (or One Meal Per Day)

Some people only eat one meal per day while on a cleanse. In that case simply fast until you have your one meal.

24 hour fasts have the same benefits as Intermittent Fasting - you're simply extending the fast as long as possible each day.

A study by David Sabatini, an MIT professor of biology and member of the Whitehead Institute for Biomedical Research and the Koch Institute discovered that fasting induces a metabolic switch in the intestinal stem cells, from utilizing carbohydrates to burning fat. Switching these cells to fatty acid oxidation enhanced their function significantly.

"Intestinal stem cells are responsible for maintaining the lining of the intestine, which typically renews itself every five days. When an injury or infection occurs, stem cells are key to repairing any damage. As people age, the regenerative abilities of these intestinal stem

cells decline, so it takes longer for the intestine to recover.

Intestinal stem cells are the workhorses of the intestine that give rise to more stem cells and to all of the various differentiated cell types of the intestine. Notably, during aging, intestinal stem function declines, which impairs the ability of the intestine to repair itself after damage," Yilmaz says. "In this line of investigation, we focused on understanding how a 24-hour fast enhances the function of young and old intestinal stem cells."[8]

Since the digestive tract is the prime focus of detox and juice cleanses, this discovery by Sabatini, et al, is a game changer in terms of how to *actually* rejuvenate intestinal health.

Thus, the occasional 24 hour fast, even outside of your typical cleanse, can be considered as something you would implement even as often as weekly. Simply plan and eat all of your calories in a single meal and fast until the next day.

Type 3: 3 Day Fast

Intermittent fasting can be practiced most days of the week. In fact, there are many people who do it daily on a continuous basis - even outside of a cleanse or detox regimen.

24-hour fasts can be done once or twice weekly on a continuous basis - and this is a good aim for a short term cleanse as well.

If, however, you want to get the most out of your detox, and you're only going to do it for 5-7 days, then you could do a 24 hour fast for the entire cleanse.

The 3 day fast, on the other hand, is a little more intensive and should probably only be practiced once every month.

Clinical trials reveal that cutting back on food for just 5 days a month could help prevent or treat age-related illnesses like diabetes and cardiovascular disease. Previous studies in rodents and humans have suggested that periodic fasting can reduce body fat, cut insulin levels, and provide other benefits.[18]

With all the detox and healing benefits, a 3 day fast may be THE best way to start a cleanse or detox.

A little planning makes a 3 day fast a lot easier. We like to start on either a Sunday or a Monday to kick the week off right.

Try to plan your cleanse outside of any weeks you might have work or family obligations.

Make sure to clear your house of any tempting foods or goodies that would seriously test your will power.

Not that fasting for 3 days is particularly hard. In fact, the biggest issue for many people is the boredom and having to find ways to fill all the extra time now that you're not spending hours a day thinking about food, making the food, then eating the food.

So, if you want to kickstart your cleanse, start right out the gate with a 3 day fast. Then transition into carnivore eating for the remainder of the days.
A week-long cleanse with fasting might look like this:

Sunday: Day 1 of a 3 day fast: drink water freely.
Monday: Day 2 of a 3 day fast: drink water freely.
Tuesday: Day 3 of a 3 day fast: here you can break the fast at dinnertime or continue until Wednesday morning depending on how you feel.
Wednesday: Break the fast with some meat or eggs for your first meal. Eat meat or eggs when hungry for the rest of the day. Drink water freely.

Thursday: Intermittent fast until noon or 1pm. Eat 3 meals of meat before 8pm. Drink water freely.
Friday: Intermittent fast until noon or 1pm. Eat 3 meals of meat before 8pm. Drink water freely.
Saturday: Intermittent fast until noon or 1pm. Break your fast with meat. Return to your normal eating pattern with Dinner.

Fasting Summary

No need to stress or freak out about fasting. No need to make it complicated. If you're not hungry, fast. If you're between meals, do not snack, just fast.

Now you know that if you skip a meal, it can actually be very healing. So try to work some fasting into your Cleanse.

Intermittent fast daily.

24 hour fast once per week.

3-5 Day fast once per month at the most, or once every 3 months at a minimum.

This is the optimum schedule to get the most benefits from fasting with the least amount of time and effort. The healing and detoxification benefits are just too great to ignore.

Carnivore Cleanse Part 2: Beef, Fish and Eggs

We discussed earlier how vegetables are not the cure-all fountain of youth they've been made out to be.They may have benefits when added to a healthy protein-rich diet - but they do come with a chemical burden that may not be appropriate during a detox program.

Protein rich diets are consistently found to have health-boosting benefits. Meat contains all the vitamins and minerals needed for robust health (as it should since it contains all the nutrients to maintain a living animal) while also being easy to digest.

Maybe this shocks some of you. There are plenty of horror stories to be found online about "undigested meat after bowel movement" or someone trying to tell you that it takes day for meat to digest and it instead 'rots' in your intestines.

NOTHING COULD BE FURTHER FROM THE TRUTH!

The fact is that meat is fully digested by the strong acidity of the stomach. And that acid is strong because it is designed to fully digest proteins.

A cow has 4 stomachs and a stomach acid pH of 5.7 in order to digest plants and vegetable matter.[19]

A lion has one stomach and a stomach acid pH between 1 and 3 to digest meat.

Humans have one stomach and a stomach acid pH of about 1.5. Even more acidic than some carnivores![20]

"It is interesting to note that humans, uniquely among the primates so far considered, appear to have stomach pH values more akin to those of carrion feeders than to those of most carnivores and omnivores. " Beasley, DeAnna E., et al. "The evolution of stomach acidity and its relevance to the human microbiome." *PloS one* 10.7 (2015): e0134116.

There is an amazing blog with a gentleman's firsthand experience after an intestinal transplant who spent months with a jejunostomy, watching the contents of his stomach drain directly into a bag:

"Can Humans Digest Meat?"

"Because I had such an extremely short bowel, my output was very high because no absorption had taken place. *I was fed and hydrated by infusion and could literally live without eating or drinking at all.* Because of my excessive output, we had to make a rig that had a hose extending from the ostomy bag that drained into a one gallon jug. Often the hose would get clogged and my wife or sister would have to use a coat hanger wire to unplug it. Now if vegan pseudoscience is right, we would suspect that the hose was being plugged by pieces of meat.

"Never once did we see any solid chunks of meat. I became so curious about this that I once swallowed the largest chunk of meat I could possibly get down without choking. Because of the shortness of my bowel, it only took about twenty minutes for my stomach to empty into the ostomy. Better than two hours later, there were no signs of any meat chunks. **What was always clogging the ostomy tube were pieces of vegetables that were not fully chewed.**

"Entire pieces of olive, lettuce, broccoli florets, grains and seeds were found. Yet, large pieces of fat were never witnessed. As a matter of fact, all the fat from the meat was already emulsified by the bile into solution. Over time, fat would coagulate on the side walls of the ostomy bag, but never were there any solid pieces observed."

(http://roarofwolverine.com/archives/412)

So. If you really want to 'cleanse' your intestines, rest your digestive tract, and start healing, animal protein (meat) is what you want to eat.

Simple cuts of minimally processed meat, fish, and eggs are some of the cleanest, least-adulterated superfoods you can eat - IF you buy the right ones.

So what we recommend for your Carnivore Cleanse is simple: meat (beef, buffalo, venison, lamb, or goat), fish (salmon or cod), and free-range eggs.

No pork or chicken though for a simple reason: it is almost impossible to find natural free-range pork and chicken. Small amounts of both are fine for your normal diet outside of a cleanse, but while you're trying to detox, try to stick to ruminant (animals that eat grass) meat.

Whatever meat you choose, it must be grass-fed and grass-finished.

It should also be minimally processed. This means steaks and simple cuts, no ground/minced or processed meats such as sausage, bacon, or hotdogs.

We also recommend fish, and to keep it simple, we recommend only two kinds: alaskan wild caught Salmon, and wild caught Cod. Avoid all farmed fish at all costs.

Both of these fish are very clean if wild caught and contain healthy fatty acids along with their protein. Avoid any fish that says "product of china" or "product of vietnam" on the back. Those are often treated with Polyphosphates, which are used to hold water in the fish during shipping overseas for processing and again when shipped back to that States.

The last source of food we recommend is eggs. But it can be a little more challenging to find good, clean eggs. If you are going to eat eggs, **only do so if you can find "Pasture Raised" eggs**. Cage-free only means that chickens are crammed into a coop rather than in a cage. Free-range means there may be 2 square feet per chicken and perhaps a door open to the outside but these chickens rarely see the sun or sky and primarily eat corn and soy-based meal.

The organic label means nothing when it comes to eggs (or chicken) because only by providing the chickens with organic grains can they claim 'organic'. But healthy eggs (with just as much omega-3 fats as fish) will only come from chickens that are able to run around outside and eat bugs. It is the insects they eat that give them the good fats for the eggs.

Pasture-Raised chickens are given at least 108 square feet outdoors and are free to eat some feed and lots of grass, bugs, worms and anything else they can find in the dirt. They are often let out of the barns first thing in the morning and spend the day outside.

Pasture-raised hens also produce healthier eggs. Penn State researchers found that one pasture-raised egg contains twice as much omega-3 fat, three times more vitamin D, four times more vitamin E and seven times more beta-carotene than eggs from hens raised on traditional feed.[21]

Another quick note about eggs. For years we've been led to believe that eggs have too much fat and will cause heart disease. But I there have been many studies of the last 10 years that show that not only do they not cause heart disease, they are healthier to eat than wheat, grains, and sugar.

Eating up to 12 eggs a week does not increase cardiovascular risk factors in people with prediabetes or type 2 diabetes, new research finds – despite conflicting dietary advice continuing around the world. University of Sydney researchers aim to help clear up conflicting dietary advice around egg consumption, as a new study finds eating up to 12 eggs per week for a year did not increase cardiovascular risk factors in people with pre-diabetes and type 2 diabetes.[22]

If 12 eggs per week is healthy in sick diabetics, they are certainly healthy foods to eat during a cleanse.

In fact, in a study of 500,000 people, the more eggs you eat, the lower your risk of heart disease! Compared with non-consumers, daily egg consumption was associated with lower risk of CVD (11% lower risk). Corresponding multivariate-adjusted HRs (95% CI) for IHD (ischemic heart disease), MCE (major coronary events), haemorrhagic stroke and ischaemic stroke were 12%, 14%, 26% and 10% respectively.[23]

Eggs are pretty much the original superfood!

<u>Beef, Fish, and Eggs Summary</u>

Outside of your fasting window, eat one to three meals of either meat, fish, or eggs. Try to find grass-fed meat, wild-caught fish, and pasture-raised eggs.

Eat until full, then stop and begin your fast until the next day. Drink water freely.

By only choosing meat, fish, and eggs that are raised as close to wild as possible, we can get the foods we have evolved to thrive on. And as we've mentioned, we believe in animal welfare, sustainability, and humane farming and fishing practices - luckily those practices also result in the most healthy meats and foods.

Carnivore Cleanse Part 3: Water

Water is the third part of the Carnivore Cleanse and is the last ingredient you need for a proper detox.

Good clean water is an absolute requirement for robust health. Water is used in nearly every process that occurs in your body and is critical for detoxification.

One of the reasons we're against the idea of a vegetable or fruit cleanse is that vegetables or fruits introduce fiber, pesticides, sugar (which feeds bad gut bacteria), and natural plant and fruit antinutrients that are counterproductive for a true cleanse.

Water, on the other hand, ideally contains just water (and maybe some trace minerals) and works with your body to remove those pesticides, heavy metals, irritants and antinutrients. But in order for it to do its job, your water must also be clean and pure of contaminants.

True detoxification of your body is done by your liver and your kidneys as long as they have an adequate supply of fluid. Therefore, proper hydration is critical.

First, we need to address the fact that most tap water is contaminated with all kinds of….crap. You can find the complete list at the EPA at

https://www.epa.gov/ground-water-and-drinking-water/national-primary-drinking-water-regulations

But it might surprise you to know that small amounts of these contaminants are found in most public water systems:

Asbestos
Cyanide
Mercury
Herbicides, industrial chemical runoff, insecticides, petroleum refinery discharge
Glyphosate
And many, *many* more

Read this excerpt from Vice online:

"Your body doesn't look at pharmaceuticals as something you're taking to help you; it looks at them as foreign chemicals and many of them are not completely degraded in the body," explains Edward Furlong, a research chemist with the US Geological Survey in Denver who has conducted extensive research on this issue. What's more, prescription drugs can enter our waterways and drinking water supplies through manufacturing waste, animal excretion, runoff from animal feeding operations, or leaching from municipal landfills, according to a 2010 report from the Natural Resources Defense Council (NRDC).[24]

Here's the real shocker: The presence of pharmaceuticals is not regulated in our drinking water supply. "People may find it hard to believe, but this country still doesn't require our drinking water systems to remove prescription drugs and many other contaminants from our tap water," says Erik Olson, director of NRDC's Health program. "In the same way that many of our roads and bridges are falling apart, our drinking water systems are aging, and most use outdated treatment technologies that don't remove a wide variety of today's contaminants, ranging from pharmaceuticals to many industrial chemicals and pesticides. We're not optimistic that the new EPA [under the current administration] will do much about this."

These pharmaceutical agents include analgesic, antibiotic, anticoagulant, antidepressant, antihistamine, and antihypertensive drugs, hormones (from oral contraceptives and hormone-therapy), and muscle relaxants, among others. Lithium (used to treat bipolar disorder), carbamazepine (an analgesic/anticonvulsant), metoprolol (an antihypertensive), and buproprion (an antidepressant) were the most frequently detected drugs in the water samples after treatment.

Experts are concerned about the long-term effects from repeated exposure because "they have the potential to bio-accumulate and be toxic to humans," according to a scientific review by researchers at Anglia Ruskin University in Cambridge, UK.[25]

(https://tonic.vice.com/en_us/article/d7bp8k/there-are-drugs-in-your-drinking-and-bottled-water)

So we know we need water but we also now know that our tap water is full of chemicals and pharmaceuticals. And unfortunately, a lot of bottled water is just repackaged tap water. About 40 percent of bottled water IS regular tap water, which may or may not have received any additional treatment. In fact, most municipal tap water must adhere to stricter purity standards than the bottled water industry.[26,27]

In addition, there are a lot of chemicals that can be leached from plastic bottles and jugs. We've all seen the reports of BPA which mimics estrogen in the body. What you may not know is that plastics labelled 'BPA-free' simply replaced the BPA with other chemicals (BPB, pthalates, and others).

One such chemical is fluorene-9-bisphenol, or BHFP for short. Frequently used in water bottles that are BPA-free, chinese researchers found that in mice, BHFP caused uterine problems and miscarriages.[28]

Unfortunately, that means that bottled or jugged water from the store is not ideal for our cleanse. Even distilled water, which is normally devoid of contaminants has probably leeched hormone disrupting chemicals from its plastic container.

The exception here would be if you can somehow find a good glass bottled water. Look for glass bottled water that says "reverse osmosis filtered". Buying glass bottled water is likely to be expensive but if you're only buying for a one or two week cleanse it might be a viable option for you.

Plan for a minimum of 1 gallon of water per day (per person doing the cleanse - it's always nice when you can do a cleanse with someone for mutual support!).

To get the cleanest water possible at home requires a reverse osmosis system. These can be found at all major home improvement stores as well as Costco and online at Amazon. They do require a bit more work in terms of installation but reverse osmosis is top of line in terms of clean water. Prices can range from

$150 and up and they do usually have a pre-filter which needs to be changed regularly but don't let this scare you - if you can afford to get a reverse osmosis system we highly recommend you do so.

We realize, however, that not everyone can afford to spend $150+ for a filter and installation.

For most people the most practical and economical path to clean water will be an NSF certified faucet filter from either PUR or Brita. These are affordable and easy to install by yourself. And while they won't get your water as clean as a reverse osmosis system, they will remove heavy metals, industrial pollutants and pesticides as well as pharmaceuticals. You can see the list of contaminants PUR can filter at:

https://www.pur.com/why-pur/faucet-filter-comparison

We have no relationship with either PUR or Brita and are not being paid to promote them - we simply recommend them as brand leaders that are easy to find and use.

One last note about water: once you've set up your home water filter, pick up a reusable water bottle so you can take your filtered water with you. Pick one made of either stainless steel or glass - not only will you reduce pollution caused by single-use plastic water bottles, you'll avoid contaminating your nice clean filtered water. This is a great way to ensure you have access to clean, filtered water while on the go, at the gym, or while at work.

<u>How much water should you drink:</u>

You should aim for ½ your bodyweight in pounds of ounces of water per day as a **minimum**. Once you meet that minimum amount, drink as much as you like. Thirst is often confused for hunger so when you think you're getting hungry, always drink a glass of water first.

So for a 100 lb woman - you'd be looking at 50 ounces *minimum* daily.

For a 200 lb man, drink a *minimum* of 100 ounces per day.

Water Summary

Make it a priority to purchase some type of water filter for your home and at least one reusable water bottle made from either stainless steel or glass for on the go.

Water is the cornerstone of good health so it only makes sense to have the cleanest water possible and have it ready to drink whenever you're thirsty or feeling hunger pangs between meals.

About Fiber

The question of fiber always comes up when talking about the carnivore cleanse. Obviously if you're just eating meat and drinking water you're not eating any vegetable fiber.

In a traditional juice cleanse - where fruits and vegetables are juiced and the fiber discarded (as done by all juicers) - there is little to no fiber anyway.

But isn't fiber supposed to be healthy?!?!

Believe it or not, for patients with bowel diseases such as Irritable Bowel Syndrome (IBS), Crohn disease, ulcerative colitis, bowel obstruction, diverticulitis, pre- and/or post-abdominal surgery, and other gastrointestinal or inflammatory disorders such as in patients with infectious gastrointestinal disease a LOW or NO fiber diet is increasingly recommended as the first-line therapy![28]

That means a *low* fiber diet is the first step in healing these debilitating intestinal issues!

If low fiber diets are used to heal real, clinical, debilitating diseases, imagine how healing they must be for a cleanse - a provent opportunity for your digestive tract to rest and rejuvenate!!!

Low fiber is also often thought to be associated with constipation but clinical studies have actually shown the opposite to be true:

In a study published by the World Journal of Gastroenterology:

"For no fiber, reduced fiber and high fiber groups, respectively, symptoms of bloating were present in 0%, 31.3% and 100% ($P < 0.001$) and straining to pass stools occurred in 0%, 43.8% and 100% ($P < 0.001$).

CONCLUSION: Idiopathic constipation and its associated symptoms can be effectively reduced by stopping or even lowering the intake of dietary fiber."[29]

In the study, the NO fiber diet was associated with zero bloating and zero constipation, leading the researchers to recommend stopping the intake of dietary fiber. On the other hand, there are actual reports of hospitalizations due to intestinal blockages due to too much fiber.

Raw vegan diets consist of nothing but vegetables, which obviously contain huge amounts of indigestible vegetable fiber. In fact, this large amount of fiber is often considered a benefit of a vegan diet. What they don't tell you though, is that these fibers can create what are called phytobezoars in the intestines.

A phytobezoar is a type of trapped mass in the gastrointestinal system that is made up indigestible plant material, such as fibres, skins and seeds. And people worry about meat getting stuck!

Phytobezoars can become large enough to cause bowel obstructions in people who eat raw vegan diets.[29]

And with the increasing misinformation about veganism, parents are mistakenly feeding their growing children raw vegan diets and no the infants too are suffering from bowel obstructions due to large amounts of indigestible plant fiber![30,31,32]

So, if you're worried about the lack of fiber in the Carnivore Cleanse, don't be - the lack of vegetable fiber will be healing.

Cleanse Length

How long you continue a Cleanse depends entirely on both how you feel during the Cleanse, as well as how much healing you are looking for.

A big advantage of the Carnivore Cleanse is that you can continue it indefinitely. If you have extra weight to lose, the Cleanse can be used for extended periods as a great weight loss diet. If you are already of a normal weight and are just looking to either Cleanse for longevity and preventative reasons, then one or two weeks a few times a year should suffice.

We recommend you try either a 3 day or 5 day cleanse if you are new to either cleanses or fasting.

If you've done cleanses in the past and are familiar and comfortable with longer durations, a 7 to 14 day cleanse is a great way to get really deep healing.

The next several pages are show examples of what a 3, 5, 7, and 14 day Carnivore Cleanse schedule might look like.

Feel free to move things around as you see fit.
The meals are all interchangeable - simply eat
as much as you need to feel full! Simple!

3 Day Carnivore Cleanse for Beginners

Day	Day One	Day Two	Day Three
Breakfast	Scrambled Eggs	Scrambled Eggs	Scrambled Eggs
Lunch	Salmon	Hamburger	Cod Filets
Dinner	Ribeye Steak	Salmon Steak	Ribeye Steak

3 Day Carnivore Cleanse with Daily Intermittent Fasting

Day	Day One	Day Two	Day Three
Morning	Fast Until Noon	Fast Until Noon	Fast Until Noon
Meal 1	Scrambled Eggs	Ribeye Steak	Hamburger
Meal 2	Ribeye Steak	Salmon	Hard Boiled Eggs
Meal 3	Cod Filets (optional if still full from Meal 2)	Hard Boiled Eggs (optional if still full from Meal 2)	Salmon (optional if still full from Meal 2)
7:00pm	Stop eating for the day	Stop eating for the day	Stop eating for the day

5 Day Cleanse with a Single 24 Hour Fast

Day	Day One	Day Two	Day Three	Day Four	Day Five
Break-fast	Fast all day	Scrambled Eggs	Hardboiled Eggs	Fast Until Noon	Fast Until Noon
Lunch	Fast all day	Hamburger	Salmon	Cod Filets	Salmon
Dinner	Fast all day	Ribeye Steak	Ribeye Steak	Hamburger	Ribeye Steak

7 Day Cleanse with a 3 Day Fast

Day	One	Two	Three	Four	Five	Six	Seven
Break-fast	Fast all day	Fast all day	Fast all day	Scrambled Eggs	Hard boiled Eggs	Salmon	Scrambled Eggs
Lunch	Fast all day	Fast all day	Fast all day	Salmon	Ham-burger	Ribeye Steak	Salmon
Dinner	Fast all day	Fast all day	Fast all day	Ribeye Steak	Cod Filet	Cod Filet	Hamburger

14 Day Cleanse with 24 Hour Fasts and Intermittent Fasting

Day	1	2	3	4	5	6	7
Break-fast	Fast all day	Fast all day	Fast all day	Scramble Eggs	Fast until Noon	Fast until Noon	Scramble Eggs
Lunch	Fast all day	Fast all day	Fast all day	Salmon	Scramble Eggs	Cod	Salmon
Dinner	Fast all day	Fast all day	Fast all day	Ribeye Steak	Cod Filet	Salmon	Ham-burger

Day	8	9	10	11	12	13	14
Break-fast	Fast all day	Scramble Eggs	Fast until Noon	Fast until Noon	Fast until Noon	Fast until Noon	Fast until Noon
Lunch	Fast all day	Cod Filet	Scramble Eggs	Salmon	Ham-burger	Ribeye Steak	Salmon
Dinner	Fast all day	Ribeye Steak	Salmon	Ribeye Steak	Cod Filet	Salmon	Ham-burger

Shopping Guide

Remember that when you eat, eat until you're satisfied. Then stop eating, and do not snack until either your next scheduled meal or you are hungry again (but remember to drink water freely!).

If you follow this recommendation, then obviously not only will the amount of beef, fish, and eggs you need to buy vary - it will vary day to day and person to person.

Accordingly, the following shopping lists are only a guideline to help get you started.

In the beginning, you may even want to buy a little extra in case there are days you are extra hungry. It's better to have a little extra on hand and ready to eat than be tempted or forced to stop your cleanse early.

Typically, we would see a 200 lb man eat something like this at one sitting for each entree:

Steak: 1 Steak, approx 1 lb
Fish: 2 Salmon filets, approx ½ lb
Eggs: 4-6 eggs
Hamburger: 2-3 x ¼ lb patties

Using those estimates as a starting point, for the 3 day cleanse as laid out in the previous chapters, this would be your shopping list:

1 dozen eggs
1 lb ground beef (85/15)
2 x Ribeye steaks - approx 1 lb each
4 x Salmon filets - approx 1-1.5 lbs total
2 x Cod filet - approx ½ lb total

For the 5 Day Cleanse with a Single 24 Hour Fast:

1 dozen eggs
1 lb ground beef (85/15)
3 x Ribeye steaks - approx 1 lb each
2 x Salmon filets - approx 1 lbs total
1 x Cod filets - approx ⅓-½ lb total

For the 7 Day Cleanse with a 2 Day Fast:

2 dozen eggs
1 lb ground beef (85/15)
2 x Ribeye steaks - approx 1 lb each
3 x Salmon - approx 1.5 - 2 lbs total
2 x Cod filets approx 1 lb total

For the 14 Day Cleanse with 24 Hour Fasts and Intermittent Fasting:

3 dozen eggs

1.5 lb ground beef (85/15)
4 x Ribeye steaks - approx 1 lb each
7 x Salmon - approx 4-5 lbs total
4 x Cod filets - approx 2 lbs total

Saving money on Meats and Fish

First, remember that all of these meals are interchangeable as long as you stick to Beef, Fish, and Eggs. So, if one or the other happens to be on sale, pick up as much as you can and simply have more meals of that one type.

IT IS PERFECTLY OK IF YOU EVEN JUST WANT TO EAT THE SAME MEAL EVERY DAY FOR THE ENTIRE CLEANSE.

There are many carnivore eaters who eat a ribeye steak for every meal. That's perfectly ok to do for the duration of the cleanse! Longer term, you will probably start to desire a little more variety, but there is really no nutritional requirement that says you **must** eat different animals.

Second, make use of a food vacuum sealer. When you find items on sale, stock up with as much as you can afford and vacuum seal the extras for longer term freezing. Beef and fish regularly rotate being on sale so this is a great way to take advantage of that for a long cleanse or even to stock up for your next cleanse.

Speaking of sales, we've found mygrocerydeals.com to be a great resource for finding what might be on sale in your area. You can find their website at:

https://www.mygrocerydeals.com/

Big discount store are often good places to look for bulk deals. Costco has good prices on frozen fish fillets (make sure they're labelled 'wild caught') as well as packs of steaks. This is especially cost effective if you use a vacuum sealer to freeze what you don't immediately use.

Remember to join us online as well where we share sales and deals as well as cleanse support and advice:

Join us online at:

https://www.facebook.com/groups/carnivoreplus/

After the Cleanse: What Next

One of the great advantages to the Carnivore Cleanse is that because it consists of real, whole foods, does not restrict the amount that you eat, and contains the essential proteins and fatty acids required by the human body, it is perfectly safe to consume long term.

In fact, it is perfectly suited as a weight loss diet as it completely eliminates fattening simple carbohydrates and sugar.

It is also, obviously, gluten free making it perfect for those with Crohn's or IBS.

Hopefully by this point you've tried either a 3- or 5-day cleanse and have seen firsthand how healing and detoxifying it is. If so, you should have a good idea how well it works for you individually and whether the short or longer term cleanses are a good fit.

With that experience in hand, there are several choices people make after completing their first cleanse:

1. Repeat the 3-day cleanse every week or so. This is a great way to lose weight in a rapid, but healing, fashion.
2. Move to a longer 7-, 10-, or 14-day cleanse to experience greater healing.
3. Add more fasting days to the shorter cleanses. Fasting is healing and detoxifying on its own and many people find that they can accelerate both weight loss and healing by adding more fasting (both by skipping individual meals and by adding more fasted days).
4. Repeat the 7- or 14-day cleanse continuously. This is another great way to lose weight but with a little more variety.

Additional Resources

If you'd like to learn more about the Carnivore Diet, we recommend the following articles and websites:

http://justmeat.co/
http://meatheals.com/
http://www.empiri.ca/p/eat-meat-not-too-little-mostly-fat.html
http://roarofwolverine.com/archives/412
http://www.gnolls.org/1444/does-meat-rot-in-your-colon-no-what-does-beans-grains-and-vegetables/

References

1. https://www.newscientist.com/article/2081497-women-live-longer-than-men-but-suffer-more-years-of-poor-health/
2. https://en.wikipedia.org/wiki/Obesity_in_the_United_States
3. http://news.mit.edu/2018/fasting-boosts-stem-cells-regenerative-capacity-0503
4. Syed, Fahd; Mena Gutiérrez, Alejandra; Ghaffar, Umbar (2 April 2015). "A Case of Iced-Tea Nephropathy". New England Journal of Medicine.
5. https://vitals.lifehacker.com/organic-food-has-pesticides-too-1825156951
6. Saunders, R. OBES SURG (2004) 14: 98. https://doi.org/10.1381/096089204772787374
7. https://www.ncbi.nlm.nih.gov/pubmed/28988855
8. http://news.mit.edu/2018/fasting-boosts-stem-cells-regenerative-capacity-0503
9. https://www.telegraph.co.uk/science/2016/03/12/fasting-for-three-days-can-regenerate-entire-immune-system-study/
10. https://www.ncbi.nlm.nih.gov/pmc/articles/PMC329619/
11. https://www.cell.com/cell-metabolism/fulltext/S1550-4131(18)30253-5
12. https://www.sciencedirect.com/science/article/pii/S0104423013000213
13. https://doi.org/10.18632/aging.100690
14. Alirezaei M, Kemball CC, Flynn CT, Wood MR, Whitton JL, Kiosses WB. Short-term fasting induces profound neuronal autophagy.

Autophagy. 2010;6(6):702-710. doi:10.4161/auto.6.6.12376.

15. https://www.ncbi.nlm.nih.gov/pubmed/21106691
16. https://www.ncbi.nlm.nih.gov/pubmed/19524509
17. https://www.ncbi.nlm.nih.gov/pubmed/23773064
18. http://www.sciencemag.org/news/2017/02/five-day-fasting-diet-could-fight-disease-slow-aging
19. http://www.milkproduction.com/Library/Scientific-articles/Animal-health/The-stomach-of-the-dairy-cow/
20. https://www.ncbi.nlm.nih.gov/pmc/articles/PMC4519257/
21. http://news.psu.edu/story/166143/2010/07/20/research-shows-eggs-pastured-chickens-may-be-more-nutritious
22. https://sydney.edu.au/news-opinion/news/2018/05/07/-eggs-not-linked-to-cardiovascular-risk--despite-conflicting-adv.html
23. http://heart.bmj.com/content/early/2018/04/17/heartjnl-2017-312651
24. https://www.nrdc.org/sites/default/files/dosed4pgr.pdf
25. http://www.sciencedirect.com/science/article/pii/S0165993616301479
26. https://www.motherjones.com/environment/2014/08/bottled-water-california-drought/
27. https://www.today.com/food/your-bottled-water-coming-faucet-2D80555502
28. https://www.ncbi.nlm.nih.gov/pmc/articles/PMC4642427/
29. Ho K-S, Tan CYM, Mohd Daud MA, Seow-Choen F. Stopping or reducing dietary fiber intake reduces constipation and its associated symptoms. World Journal of Gastroenterology : WJG. 2012;18(33):4593-4596. doi:10.3748/wjg.v18.i33.4593.
30. https://www.nature.com/articles/ncomms14585

31. https://link.springer.com/article/10.1007/s10140-003-0297-0
32. https://www.ncbi.nlm.nih.gov/pubmed/29760008?dopt=Abstract
33. https://sci-hub.tw/10.1136/archdischild-2018-314910

9 781720 071389